Vintage Secretions

Disclaimer

This work is a piece of medical satire intended for educational and humorous purposes for a professional audience. All images contained herein are fully de-identified and depict biological material removed from the human airway during routine medical care.

No patient names, dates, locations, identifying features, or protected health information are included. Images were collected over time and are presented without reference to specific individuals, encounters, or institutions.

This book does not represent the views of any hospital, healthcare system, employer, or affiliated organization. The author's observations reflect a personal artistic and professional perspective shaped by clinical experience.

Nothing in this work should be interpreted as medical advice, clinical guidance, or commentary on individual patients.

Reader discretion is advised.

Vintage Secretions

A GUIDE TO RESPIRATORY OFFERINGS FROM THE CRITICALLY ILL

Lee Daniels

Published by Griffin Intellectual Property, LLC.
Author: Lee Daniels.

Author's Note

Critical care medicine occupies a strange intersection of precision, endurance, and exposure to things most people will never see. Those who work in intensive care units quickly learn that humor—particularly dark humor—is not cruelty, but a coping mechanism honed under pressure. This book is not about patients. It is about the work.

It is about the physical reality of pneumonia, aspiration, inflammation, and time. It is about the substances that accumulate quietly in the lungs while clinicians monitor numbers, titrate drips, and wait. It is about the artifacts that remain once intervention finally occurs.

By borrowing the language of wine tasting, art criticism, and luxury culture, Vintage Secretions deliberately contrasts refinement with biological chaos. The goal is not mockery, but perspective—an acknowledgment that those who care for the critically ill often process their experiences through irony, exaggeration, and shared understanding.

This book is intended for clinicians, nurses, respiratory therapists, and others who already understand the cost of this work. If it makes you laugh, pause, or feel momentarily unsettled, then it has succeeded.

Contents

Twin Offerings

Name:	Twin Offerings
Describing Term:	Bifurcated, Mucohemorrhagic, Structurally Ambitious
Likely Producer:	Staphylococcus aureus
Supporting Cast:	E. coli and opportunistic anaerobes
Environmental Influence:	Prolonged mechanical ventilation, positional neglect, and enough airway residence to develop opinions

The presentation immediately suggests curation rather than extraction: two related specimens displayed side by side on sterile gauze, the left pale, looping, and almost ornamental, the right darker, thicker, and marbled with blood. Together they read less like debris than a paired study in escalation, as though the same lung decided to offer both restraint and grievance in a single sitting.

On the nose, the left opens with warm saline and faint lactic sweetness, modest almost to the point of deceit. The right arrives with iron, inflamed tissue, and a darker organic heat, carrying the unmistakable suggestion of longer tenancy and worse intentions. The contrast is the point: one persuasive, one punitive.

The palate is divided but coherent. The left gives rope-like elasticity and easy extension before yielding; the right is denser, irregular, and clot-laced, interrupting the experience with chew, weight, and pockets of resistance. This is comparison as a clinical method.

The finish is asymmetrical. The left exits cleanly enough to encourage bad decisions, while the right lingers in metallic fragments, leaving behind the sense that extraction has occurred, but resolution has not.

Mouthfeel:	Silken on entry, punitive on finish
Structure:	Asymmetric but intentional
Harmony:	Achieved only by proximity
Extraction:	Required patience, escalation, and a second pass just to be sure

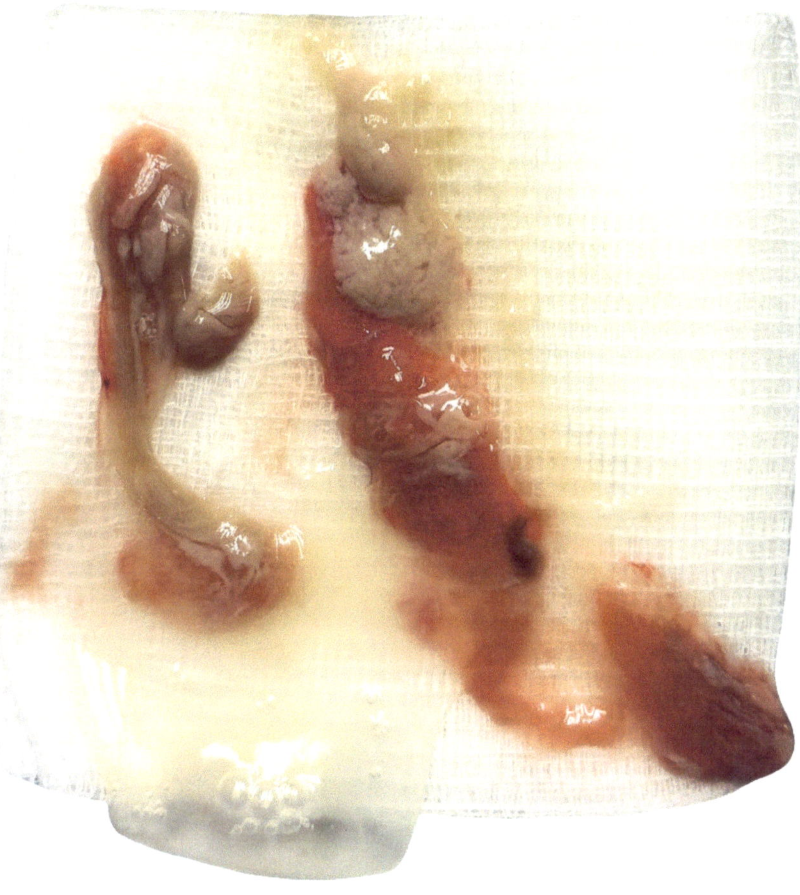

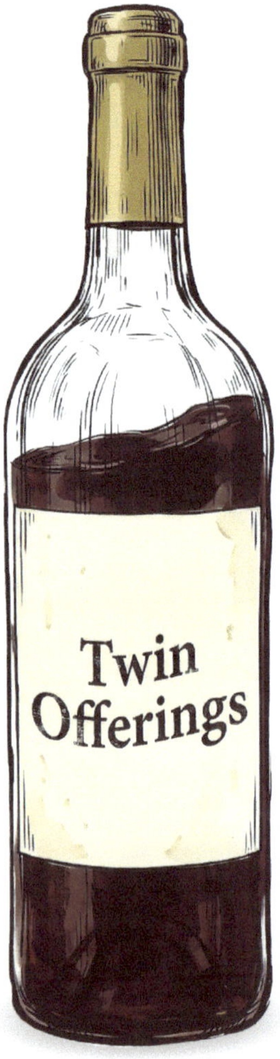

Pairs Best With

- Broad-spectrum antibiotics administered before the discussion becomes academic
- Bronchoscopy with decisive suction
- Side-by-side comparison under direct visualization

Pairs Poorly With

- Deferred bronchoscopy in the name of patience
- Any belief that symmetry implies cooperation
- The phrase, “Let’s just see how it looks tomorrow”

Brown Study

Name:	Brown Study
Describing Term:	Necrotic, Enteric-Leaning, Utterly Unrepentant
Likely Producer:	Klebsiella pneumoniae
Supporting Cast:	E. coli and anaerobes of questionable morals
Environmental Influence:	Prolonged stasis, enthusiastic aspiration, and complete disregard for pulmonary boundaries

The presentation is immediately confrontational. Thick, opaque brown effluent spreads across the gauze in an uneven glossy sheet, interrupted by bubbles that rise and hold like guilty thoughts. The color alone suggests age, density, and a degree of airway betrayal that refuses euphemism.

On the nose, there is no subtlety. Deep muddy sweetness leads, followed by damp earth, lysed tissue, and a distinctly enteric undertone that implies the specimen has forgotten where it originated. An anaerobic funk lingers at a distance and does not improve with reflection.

The palate is overwhelming. Entry is thick and coating, with immediate resistance that spreads rather than stretches. It slumps instead of elongating, pooling into itself while still refusing to disperse. This is not a strand or a cast; it is a territorial event.

The finish is long, oppressive, and personal. What remains is less a taste than an atmosphere: heavy, warm, and deeply committed to the idea that it was comfortable where it was.

Mouthfeel:	Pasty, sludgelike, accusatory
Structure:	Amorphous, overcommitted, and unconcerned with boundaries
Harmony:	None
Extraction:	Required force, patience, and emotional support

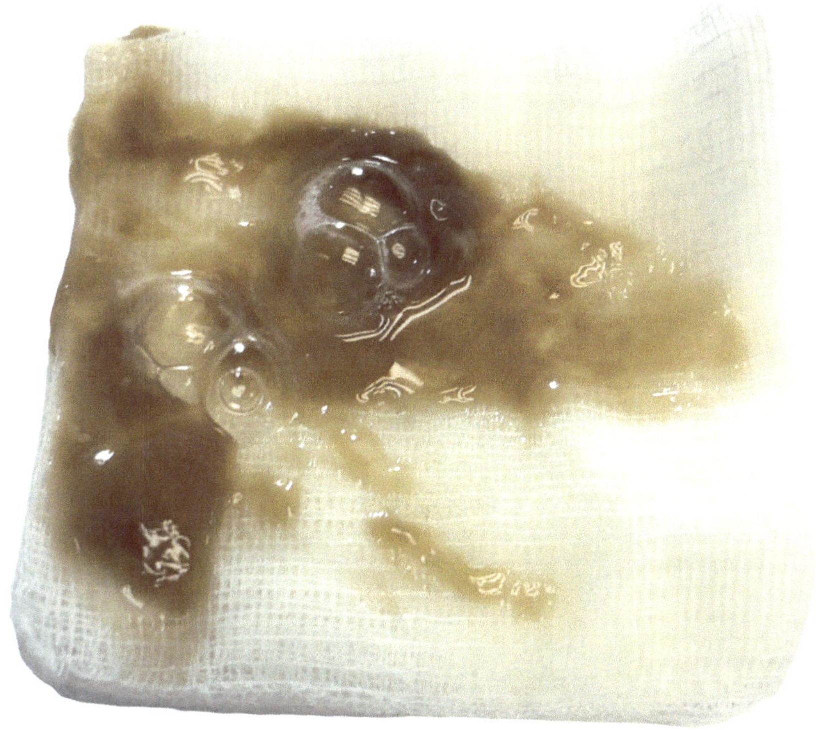

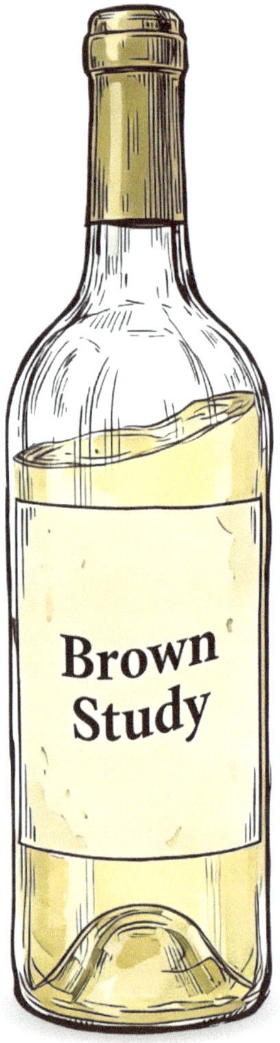

Pairs Best With

- Carbapenems
- Source control as a philosophy
- A suction canister you plan to discard immediately

Pairs Poorly With

- Resuming enteral feeds on faith alone
- Explaining aspiration away as oral secretions
- Asking, "Is that stool?"

Crimson Contamination

Name:	Crimson Contamination
Describing Term:	Hemorrhagic, High-Drama, Multiphase
Likely Producer:	Staphylococcus aureus
Supporting Cast:	Necrotizing Streptococcus, friable tissue, and recent mechanical persuasion
Environmental Influence:	Prolonged stasis, enthusiastic aspiration, and complete disregard for pulmonary boundaries

The presentation is unapologetically chaotic. Broad swaths of arterial red streak across sterile gauze, intersecting in a pattern that feels less accidental than declarative. Darker coagulated segments anchor the composition while fresher crimson smears imply movement that was recent, forceful, and unresolved.

On the nose, fresh heme dominates immediately: bright, metallic, and impatient. Beneath it sit tissue injury, inflammatory heat, and a faint sweetness that gives the whole thing the unsettling energy of active staphylococcal overperformance. Nothing about this profile reads settled.

The palate is intense from the outset. Entry is slick and hot before escalating into dense gelatinous resistance. Clotted segments provide chew and structure while surrounding fluid elements spread freely, staining everything they contact. The experience oscillates between cohesion and collapse.

The finish is abrupt in action but long in consequence. Copper, warmth, and a trace of procedural regret persist well past the point of comfort, leaving the unmistakable impression that this specimen was removed under protest and will be remembered accordingly.

Mouthfeel:	Gelatinous, streaked, confrontational
Structure:	Fragmented but forceful
Harmony:	Irrelevant
Extraction:	Required commitment and documentation afterward

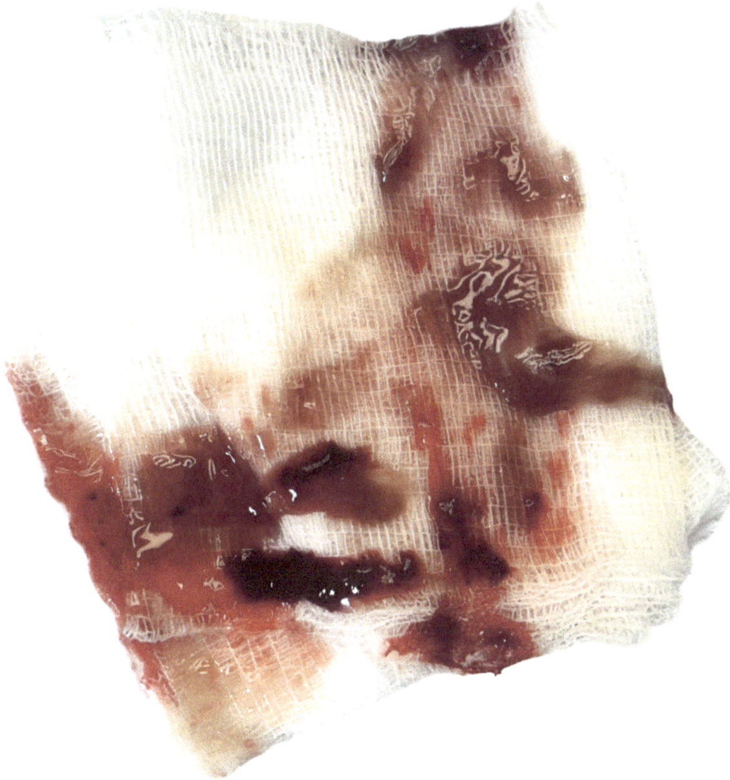

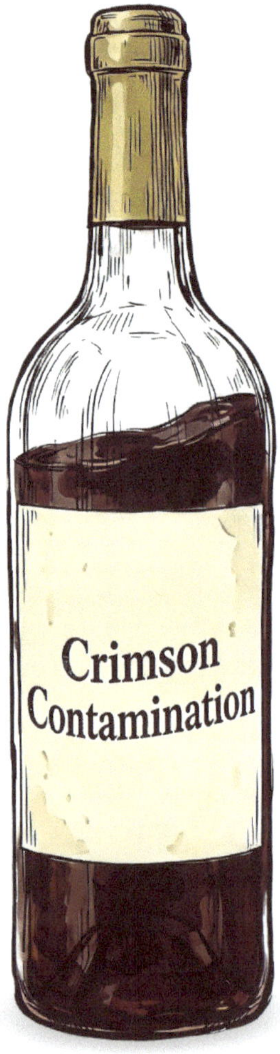

Pairs Best With

- Vancomycin administered without hesitation
- Aggressive suction and a steady hand
- A brief silence before anyone speaks

Pairs Poorly With

- Casual bronchoscopy
- Suction set one step too low
- Trainees who just wanted to take a look

Untitled (Respiratory Offering)

Name:	Untitled (Respiratory Offering)
Describing Term:	Mucoid, Expansile, Quietly Accusatory
Likely Producer:	Streptococcus pneumoniae
Supporting Cast:	Oral flora
Environmental Influence:	Time, gravity, incomplete clearance, and the slow indifference of the supine position

The presentation suggests quiet accumulation rather than urgency: a single looping specimen arranged across sterile gauze, pale amber and softly translucent, broad at its base and tapering as it extends. The form is so composed it borders on sculptural, betraying not violence but duration.

On the nose, bleached linen and warmed plastic arrive first, with saline sweetness appearing only afterward. The profile does not insist on itself. It lingers at the edge of perception, offering reminders of time, stasis, and biologic persistence rather than acute disruption.

The palate is cohesive and expansive. It spreads before it stretches, occupying space with a calm persistence that feels less resistant than inevitable. There is no dramatic fragmentation, only a quiet adaptability that allows the material to settle, extend, and re-form as needed.

The finish is prolonged but understated. A thin residual slickness remains, accompanied by the recognition that what has been removed is merely the visible portion of a longer story. The final impression is not intensity, but duration.

Mouthfeel:	Silken, cohesive, and quietly expansive
Structure:	Continuous, adaptive, and deceptively organized
Harmony:	Achieved through persistence rather than balance
Extraction:	Unresisted, but not voluntary

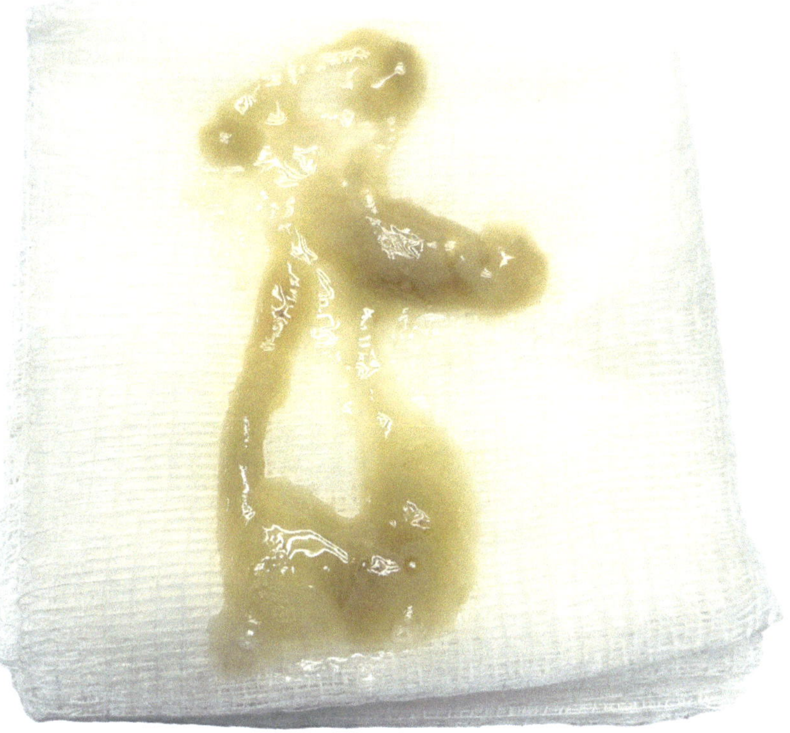

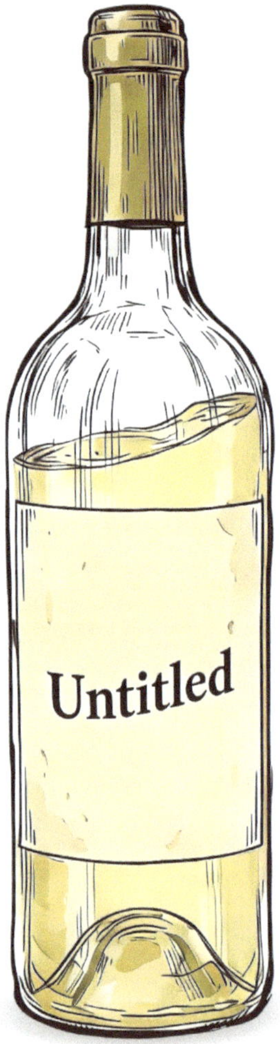

Pairs Best With

- Patient, deliberate suction
- Early recognition of accumulation
- The phrase, "There's probably more"

Pairs Poorly With

- Reassurance based on appearance alone
- Supine neglect mistaken for stability
- Any assumption that stillness implies resolution

Hooked Intent

Name:	Hooked Intent
Describing Term:	Filamentous, Mucohemorrhagic, Reluctantly Dislodged
Likely Producer:	Streptococcus pneumoniae
Supporting Cast:	Staphylococcus aureus and minor mucosal trauma
Environmental Influence:	Prolonged stasis with intermittent agitation and eventual forced removal

The presentation immediately conveys tension: a single elongated specimen curved into a distinct hook, its pale amber body interrupted by streaks of fresh crimson. The shape feels dynamic rather than passive, as though it had conformed tightly to the airway and was persuaded, not invited, to leave.

On the nose, fresh blood arrives first, with saline sweetness following behind it rather than leading. A faint warmth sits beneath the surface, subtle but unmistakable, signaling recent disturbance more than settled accumulation.

The palate is tensile and deliberate. Initial contact gives little resistance before extending into a long elastic strand that maintains continuity throughout. The blood-streaked segments interrupt with thicker, more stubborn points of adherence, suggesting that parts of this structure detached unevenly and with opinion.

The finish is unsettled rather than lingering. What remains is not slickness so much as remembered traction - the sense that this specimen left the airway in stages and left an impression where it had been.

Mouthfeel:	Elastic, cohesive, intermittently resistant
Structure:	Continuous with focal reinforcement
Harmony:	Disrupted by intervention
Extraction:	Achieved with effort and mild protest

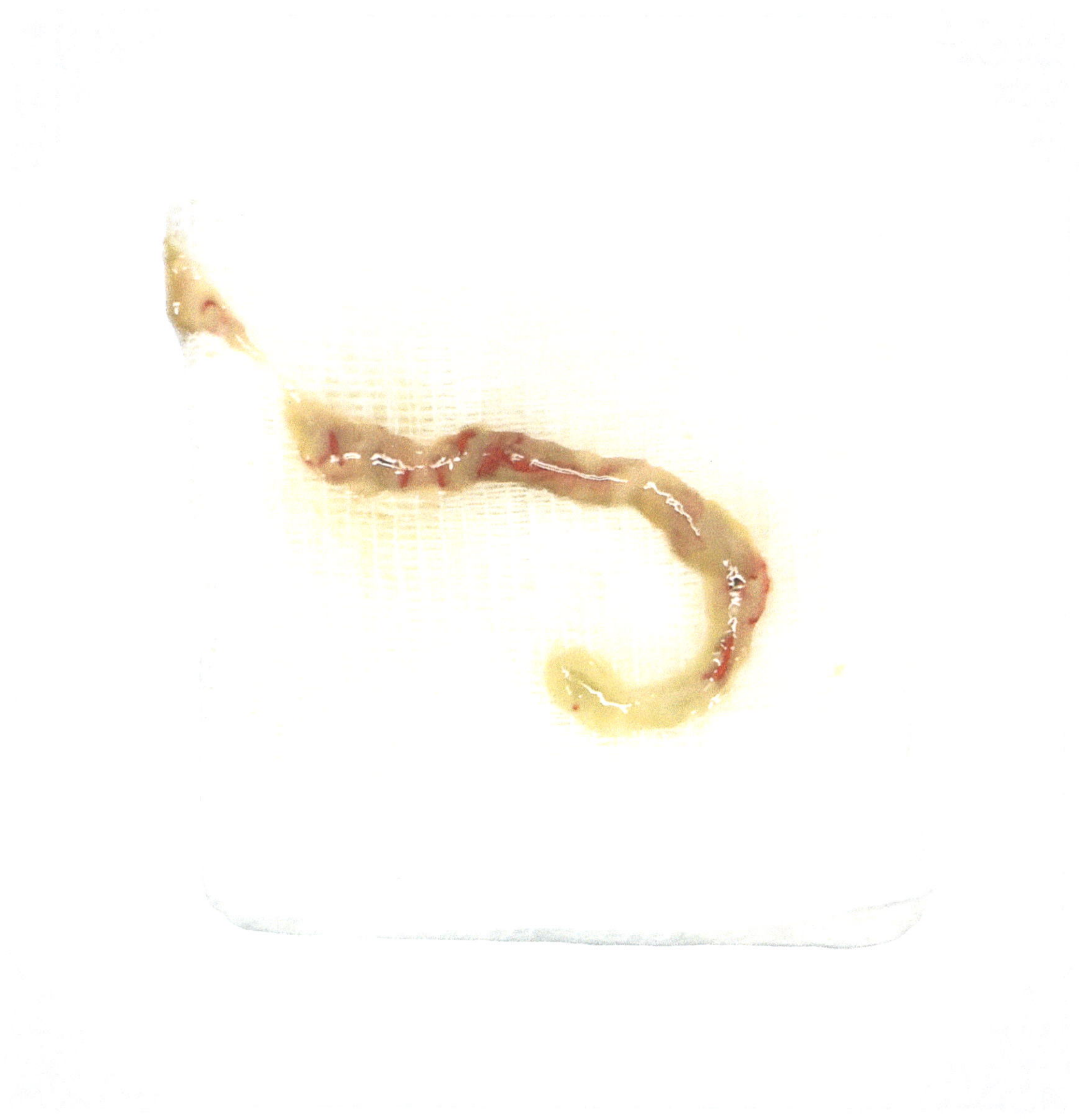

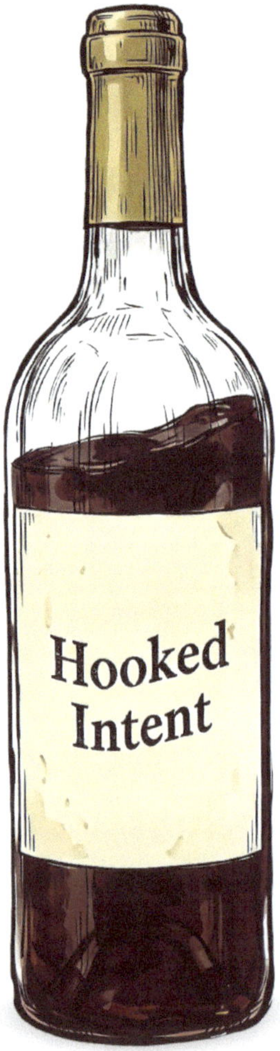

Pairs Best With

- Steady, controlled suction
- Recognition of partial adherence
- A second pass to confirm clearance

Pairs Poorly With

- Blind traction
- Ignoring blood-streaked warning signs
- Withdrawal without a second look

Pale Silk

Name:	Pale Silk
Describing Term:	Mucoid, Low-Viscosity, Socially Deceptive
Likely Producer:	Streptococcus pneumoniae
Supporting Cast:	Early Haemophilus influenzae and trace oral flora
Environmental Influence:	Early accumulation with preserved hydration and inadequate clearance

The presentation is understated at first glance: soft translucent deposits arranged in a tidy composition across sterile gauze, connected by thin glistening filaments that imply continuity beneath the surface. The coloration is pale straw to diluted ivory, clean and hydrated in a way that feels undeserved.

On the nose, there is an almost nursery-clean softness: wet paper, warm saline, and only the faintest iron beneath it. The profile remains restrained throughout, never declaring itself aggressively, which is precisely how it earns trust it has not earned.

The palate reveals the fraud. What first reads as delicate quickly proves adhesive, threading itself into continuity and reforming with irritating ease after disruption. It clings lightly but persistently, maintaining cohesion long after its appearance has promised otherwise.

The finish is quiet but recursive, the kind that makes you think it is gone until it presents again. A faint warmth remains, along with the specific irritation reserved for material that looks manageable, behaves politely, and still refuses to be finished.

Mouthfeel:	Silken, elastic, quietly defiant
Structure:	Loosely organized but highly cohesive
Harmony:	Superficial, masking underlying persistence
Extraction:	Required repeated passes despite initial optimism

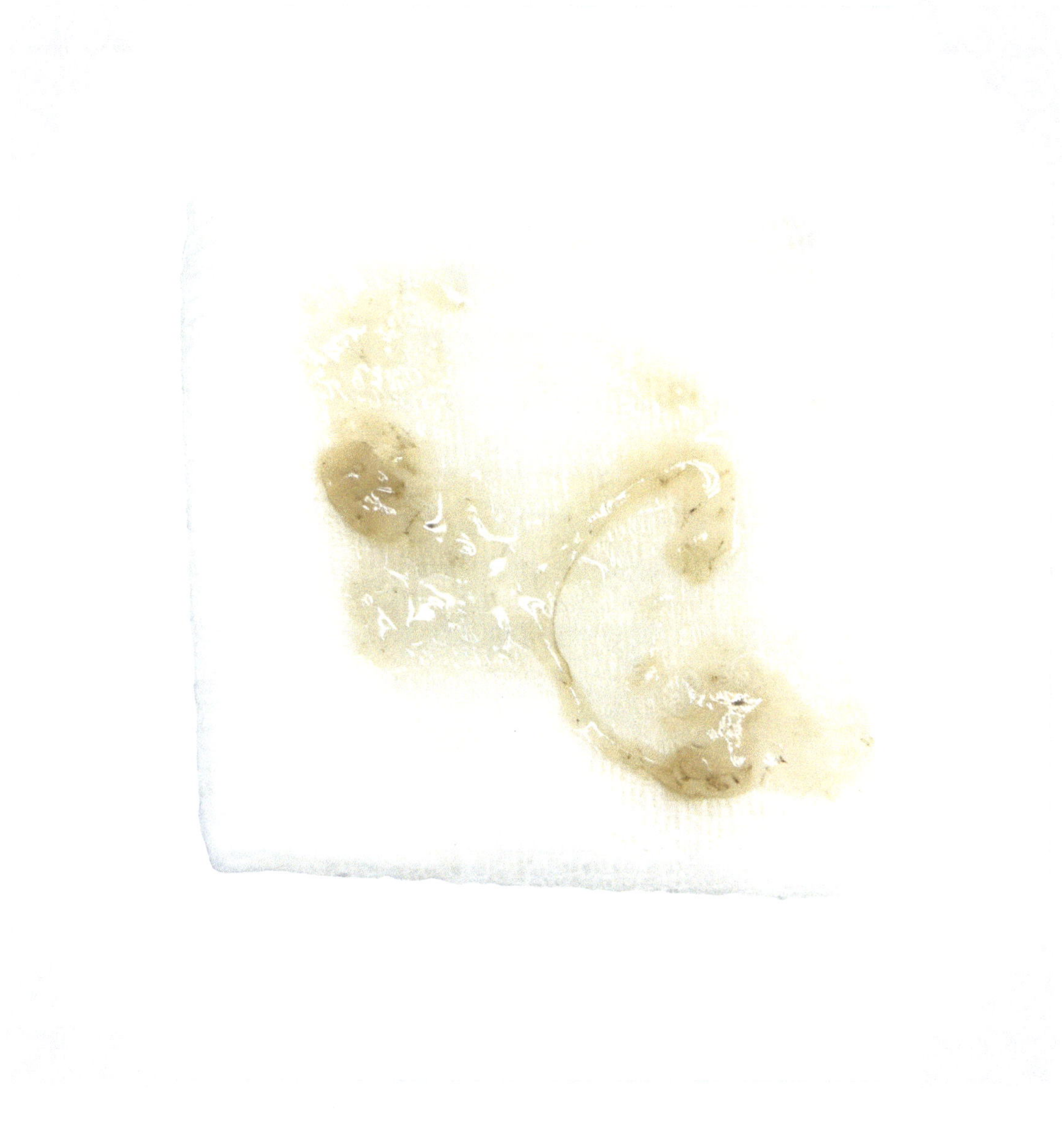

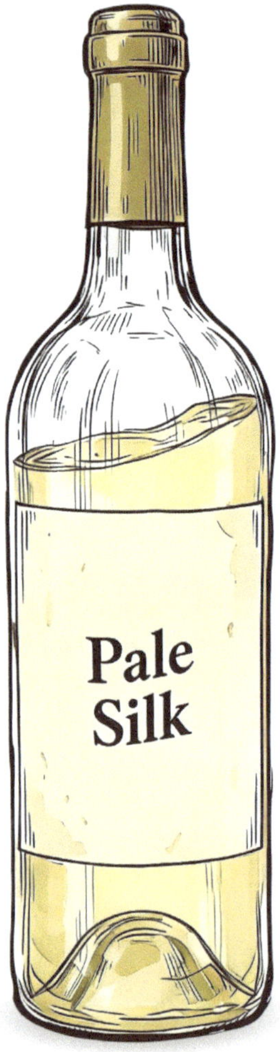

Pairs Best With

- Ceftriaxone administered early
- Gentle but persistent suction
- A willingness to reassess

Pairs Poorly With

- Single-pass satisfaction
- "That looks pretty good now"
- Chest x-rays that flatter the situation

Black Tie

Name:	Black Tie
Describing Term:	Fully Clotted, Terminally Mature
Likely Producer:	Staphylococcus aureus
Supporting Cast:	Necrosis, time, and repeated mechanical insistence
Environmental Influence:	Extended residence with zero intention of self-evacuation

The presentation is stark and unmistakable: a single elongated specimen rendered in deep obsidian red, nearly black at its core, resting against white gauze like a formal accusation. Minimal surrounding fluid reinforces the impression of completion. This is not a secretion in motion; it is a structure that has decided what it is.

On the nose, old iron dominates - dried rust, spent blood, and the dense maturity of something no longer in flux. There are no bright notes here, no sweetness, and no illusion of reversibility. The profile is heavy with age rather than activity.

The palate is immediate and unyielding. Entry offers firm resistance, with a compact cohesive structure that refuses deformation. Elasticity has been replaced entirely by resolve. This specimen does not stretch, smear, or negotiate; it exits only as a whole.

The finish is conclusive. A deep metallic warmth persists well beyond extraction, accompanied by the recognition that this represents an endpoint rather than a phase. The effect is not complexity, but completion.

Mouthfeel:	Dense, rubberized, absolute
Structure:	Fully consolidated and unyielding
Harmony:	Singular, uncompromising
Extraction:	Achieved once, correctly

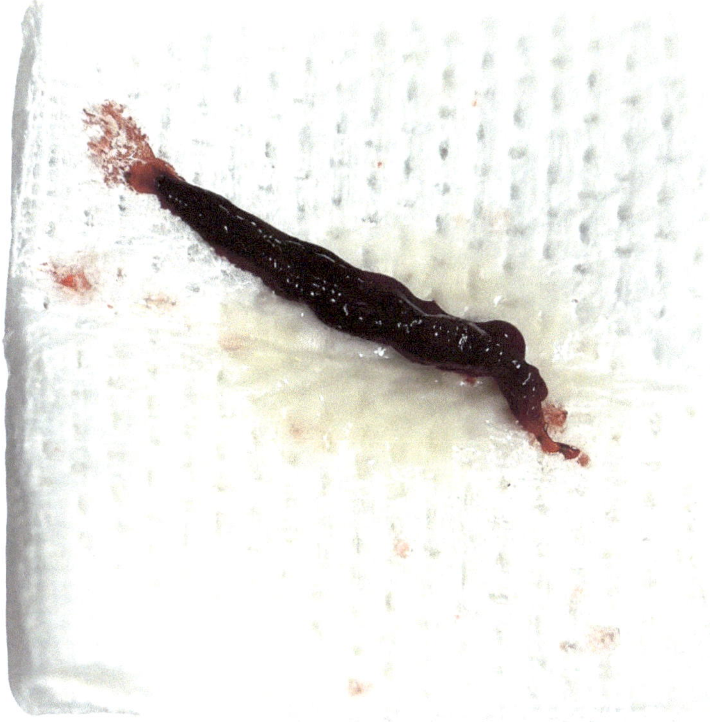

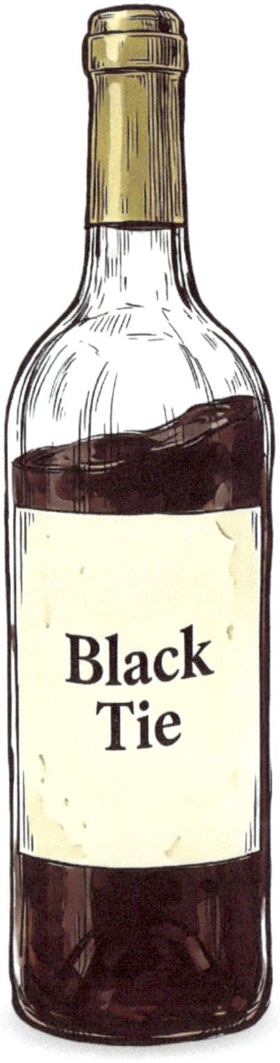

Pairs Best With

- Definitive suction under direct visualization
- Definitive source control, then antibiotics worthy of the scene
- Quiet respect from everyone in the room

Pairs Poorly With

- Anticoagulation
- Hesitation
- Anyone saying, "That's impressive" out loud

Small Regrets

Name:	Small Regrets
Describing Term:	Segmented, Mucohemorrhagic, Casually Defiant
Likely Producer:	Streptococcus pneumoniae
Supporting Cast:	Haemophilus influenzae and trace blood from repeated negotiations
Environmental Influence:	Partial clearance with persistent intent

The presentation offers a composed triptych: three discrete specimens arranged with deceptive neatness across sterile gauze, each distinct in shape yet clearly derived from a common source. The upper fragment is compact and opaque, modest in scale but firm in conviction. Below, two longer pieces extend with more confidence, their pale amber strands interrupted by darker blood-tinged nodes that mark prior adherence and eventual release.

On the nose, the profile is quieter than expected - saline first, then iron in flashes rather than a continuous note. Nothing here shouts. Instead, the aroma assembles itself gradually, suggesting persistence by accumulation rather than force.

The palate is varied across the three pieces. Each fragment behaves differently on contact: the smaller one offers dense cohesion with minimal stretch, while the longer strands extend elastically before thinning under tension. The blood-tinged nodes interrupt with brief metallic resistance, reminding the viewer that even modest specimens can argue.

The finish is cumulative rather than dramatic. A light slickness remains, accompanied by the awareness that these were merely the most cooperative portions of a larger whole. The final impression is not victory, but partial credit.

Mouthfeel:	Slick, elastic, intermittently resistant
Structure:	Fragmented but thematically consistent
Harmony:	Achieved through shared origin rather than balance
Extraction:	Achieved incrementally, never conclusively

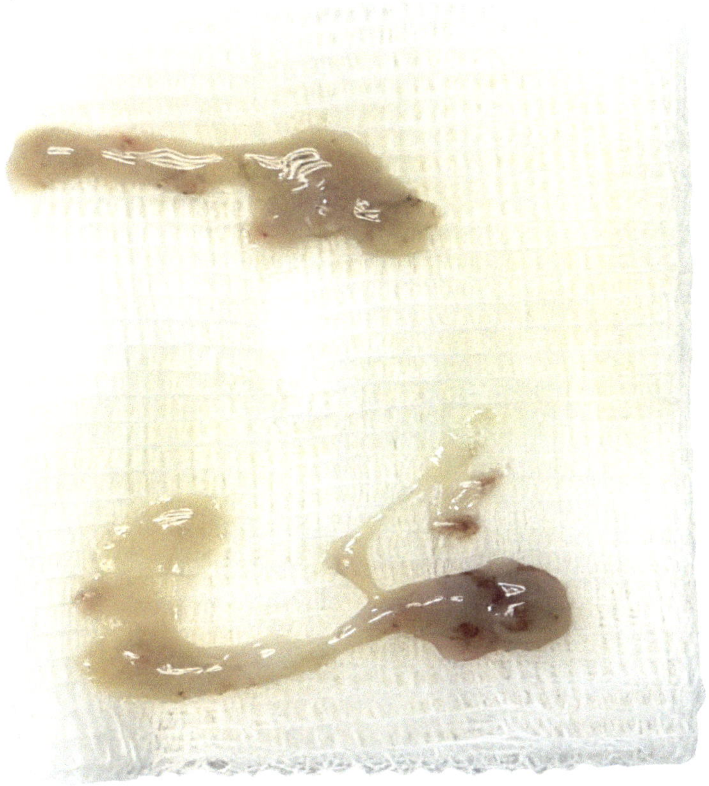

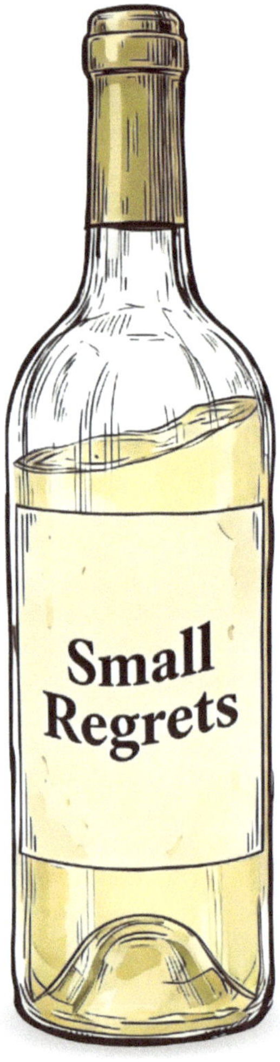

Pairs Best With

- Measured suction and patience
- Ceftriaxone administered with calm authority
- A methodical approach that assumes nothing is finished

Pairs Poorly With

- Counting pieces instead of airways
- Ignoring the smallest fragment
- Any sentence beginning with "That should be all"

Late Harvest, Ventilator Day 7

Name:	Late Harvest, Ventilator Day 7
Describing Term:	Advanced Maturity, Anaerobic-Leaning, Biofilm-Enriched
Likely Producer:	Pseudomonas aeruginosa
Supporting Cast:	Klebsiella pneumoniae and mixed flora with time-dependent evolution
Environmental Influence:	Prolonged ventilation, stasis, and microbial overachievement

The presentation reflects extended residence: a dense irregular mass suspended within a translucent amber field, its muted gray-green tones contrasting against the surrounding clarity. The specimen appears less removed than interrupted, shaped slowly by gravity, neglect, and days no one can get back.

On the nose, an immediate bloom of damp cellar and forgotten laundry emerges, assertive yet oddly restrained. Iron and anaerobic ambition follow, layered with something unmistakably hospital-adjacent, like saline left open too long under fluorescent lights. The profile feels aged rather than active.

The palate is dense and unctuous, offering a mouth-coating viscosity that speaks to prolonged stagnation. Entry is heavy and cohesive, spreading without urgency but with unmistakable weight. Mid-palate introduces a faint green bitterness suggestive of chronic aspiration and microbial complexity before settling into a thick persistent presence.

The finish is long - unforgivably long. Residual weight and damp warmth linger well beyond expectation, leaving the impression not of removal, but of interruption. What remains is not absence, but memory.

Mouthfeel:	Viscous, cohesive, and fully committed
Structure:	Mature, layered, and biofilm-informed
Harmony:	Achieved through time rather than balance
Extraction:	Delayed, but ultimately necessary

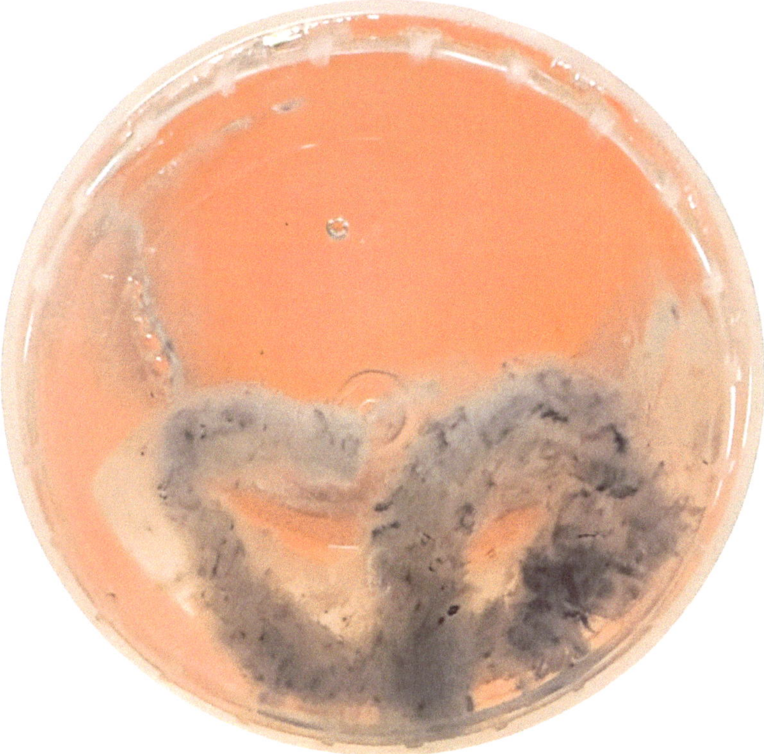

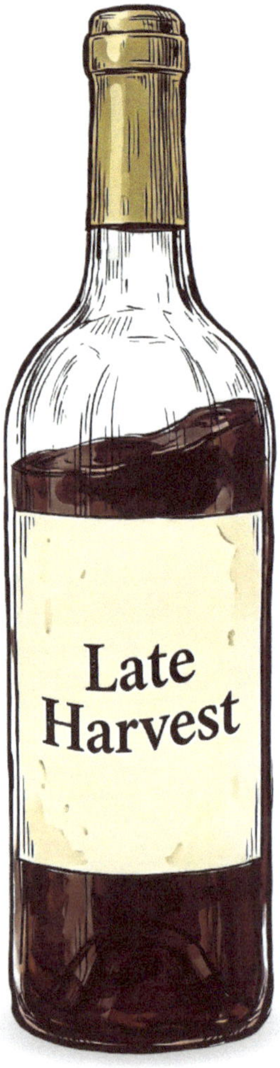

Pairs Best With

- Antipseudomonal coverage worthy of its resume
- Aggressive suction and follow-up inspection
- A healthy respect for ventilator day count

Pairs Poorly With

- Narrow coverage
- Short courses inspired by wishful thinking
- Any assumption that time improves this

About the Author

The author is a formally trained observer of human decline, having spent years cultivating a refined palate in windowless rooms illuminated exclusively by fluorescent lighting and the soft glow of monitor alarms. Their work is informed by countless overnight vigils, innumerable suction canisters, and a deeply unhealthy familiarity with secretions that were never meant to be seen, let alone contemplated.

Trained in the careful extraction and appraisal of pulmonary artifacts, the author approaches each specimen with reverence, curiosity, and a clinically inappropriate sense of wonder. Their methodology blends traditional medical practice with the sensibilities of a sommelier, an art critic, and someone who has absolutely lost the ability to be shocked.

When not cataloging the lung's most regrettable offerings, the author can be found offering unsolicited commentary on viscosity, bouquet, and "mouthfeel" to colleagues who did not ask. They are widely regarded as both deeply committed to patient care and profoundly unfit to work in polite society.

The author lives somewhere between optimism and burnout and continues to believe—against mounting evidence—that this book is an act of public service.

Afterword

A Quiet Moment Before Documentation

At the end of the day, these are just specimens. They are suctioned, collected, photographed, described, and ultimately discarded. They do not linger. They do not follow anyone home. By morning, they exist only as numbers in a note and a vague memory of resistance.

And yet.

Anyone who has done this work long enough knows that some things leave an impression. Not because they were dramatic, or catastrophic, or rare—but because they were physical reminders of time passing inside a body that could not clear itself.

This book is not an archive. It is a pause.

A brief acknowledgment that beneath ventilator settings, lab values, and progress notes, there exists a parallel record made of texture, color, volume, and effort. Most of the time, we do not name it. We simply manage it and move on.

If this collection made you laugh, it was not because the subject is trivial. If it unsettled you, it was not because it crossed a line. It did exactly what it was meant to do: reflect the strange intimacy of caring for people at their most vulnerable, through the only lens that makes sustained exposure possible.

Now the specimens are gone.

The suction is off.

The room is quiet.

It's time to document and move on.

www.ingramcontent.com/pod-product-compliance
Ingram Content Group UK Ltd.
Pitfield, Milton Keynes, MK11 3LW, UK
UKHW061414111026
15625UKWH00051B/594
9798995907930